Copyright Information

Disclaimer:

The information provided in this book is for informational and educational purposes only. The author is not a licensed medical professional, and the content is based on personal experience and informal studies in herbalism. This book is not intended to diagnose, treat, cure, or prevent any health condition. Always consult with a healthcare professional before using herbal remedies, especially if you are pregnant, nursing, or taking medication.

This book is a collaboration with
KEEP HEALTHY DZ
Design by STARTEM VISUALS

Introduction

As a woman in my late twenties, I have faced my fair share of health challenges—particularly with Irritable Bowel Syndrome (IBS), menstrual pain, and bloating. These are issues many women know all too well, and they can have a significant impact on daily life. Over the years, I've searched for ways to manage these symptoms and improve my well-being. This journey led me to a lifelong love of herbal infusions, a natural remedy that I learned about from my father. He taught me how powerful plants can be in addressing many common health issues, and, in time, I discovered that they can even help prevent others from developing.

My own experiences, combined with informal herbal studies and a course in herbalism, have allowed me to understand the healing potential of natural ingredients. This book is a reflection of the knowledge I have gained through personal experience, trial and error, and constant learning about the properties of herbs. However, it is important to note that I am not a doctor, pharmacist, or medical professional. The infusions and recipes shared in this book are based on my own experiences and the wisdom I've gathered from the world of herbalism.

Introduction

Why Infusions?

Herbal infusions are simple yet effective ways to harness the power of plants. They have been used for centuries to soothe various ailments, promote relaxation, aid digestion, and support overall well-being. What I love most about them is how they allow us to reconnect with nature, using what is readily available to restore balance in our bodies.

In this book, I focus on infusions that specifically target issues like digestive health, menstrual pain, bloating, and other challenges that many women, including myself, often face. I also highlight the scientific names of the plants used (in Latin), paying homage to their origins and traditional uses. The recipes are practical, easy to prepare, and designed to be both enjoyable and beneficial.

A Personal and Educational Journey

I want this book to be more than just a collection of recipes—it is a journey into understanding how the body and nature interact. For each herb, I provide a brief explanation of its traditional uses and how it can help support your health. My goal is for you to not only enjoy the recipes but also learn something new with each one.

Introduction

A Word of Caution

While I have seen the benefits of these infusions firsthand, I strongly recommend that you consult with a healthcare professional before trying any new herbal remedy, especially if you are pregnant, nursing, or on medication. The information in this book is not meant to replace professional medical advice.

Collaboration and Design

This book has been brought to life with the collaboration of KEEP HEALTHY DZ, who provided invaluable support in its creation, and STARTEM VISUALS, responsible for the beautiful design of the book. Their dedication has helped turn this project into a reality, and I am deeply grateful.

I hope that this collection of natural infusion recipes becomes a helpful resource for you, as it has been for me. May these remedies offer you the comfort and relief that I have experienced, and help you discover the beauty and power of plants.

How to use this book

This book has been crafted to be both educational and practical, giving you an accessible guide to natural herbal infusions that support your health and well-being. Whether you're new to herbalism or have some experience, this book is designed to be easy to follow, with straightforward instructions and helpful information about each plant used.

Here's how you can best navigate and use the book:

1. Understanding the Sections

The book is divided into different sections, each focusing on specific health issues or purposes:

• **Digestive Health:** For issues like bloating, indigestion, or discomfort related to Irritable Bowel Syndrome (IBS).
• **Menstrual and Hormonal Balance:** Infusions designed to ease menstrual cramps, support hormonal health, and soothe PMS symptoms.
• **Calming and Stress Relief:** Recipes that promote relaxation, ease anxiety, and help with better sleep.
• **Immune Support and General Wellness:** Infusions that boost your immunity and help maintain overall health.

Each section contains carefully curated recipes that are tailored to address these particular needs, using herbs with known properties that have been traditionally used for these purposes.

How to use this book

2. Recipe Layout

Each recipe is structured in a clear and simple format, allowing you to easily follow along. Here's what you'll find in every recipe:

• **Title of the Infusion:** This gives you a quick idea of what the infusion is designed for, such as "Menstrual Relief Blend" or "Digestive Calm Tea."

• **Ingredients List:** All the ingredients you will need, with their amounts specified. I've made an effort to keep the recipes simple and with easily accessible herbs.

• **Step-by-Step Instructions:** Easy-to-follow directions on how to prepare the infusion, including steeping times and any specific tips to enhance the flavor or effect.

• **Serving Size:** Information on how much the recipe yields, so you know whether it's for a single cup or a larger batch.

• **Additional Notes:** In some recipes, you'll find additional tips, such as how to adjust for taste, optional ingredients, or how to store the infusion.

How to use this book

3. Educational Insights

Next to each recipe, you'll also find **educational notes** that explain the benefits of the herbs used. This is where you can learn about each herb's traditional uses, its Latin name, and its medicinal properties. These insights help you understand not just how to make the infusion, but why it works.

For example:

- **Calendula (Calendula officinalis):** Known for its anti-inflammatory and soothing properties, great for skin and digestive health.
- **Valerian Root (Valeriana officinalis):** A natural relaxant, often used to help with anxiety and sleep issues.

4. Tailoring to Your Needs

Feel free to experiment and adjust the recipes to suit your taste and needs. Herbalism is personal, and every body responds differently to herbs. You can:

- **Mix and Match:** If you find that one herb works particularly well for you, don't hesitate to incorporate it into other blends.
- **Adjust Dosages:** Start with the recommended amounts and listen to your body. Some people may need a stronger infusion, while others might prefer a milder version.

How to use this book

5. Safety First

Herbs are powerful, and while they can offer great benefits, it's important to approach them with care:

• **Consult a Professional:** Before incorporating any new herbs into your routine, especially if you are pregnant, nursing, or taking medications, consult your healthcare provider.
• **Allergies:** Be mindful of any allergies you may have. While herbs are natural, they can still cause allergic reactions in some individuals.

6. Integrating Infusions Into Your Routine

To get the most out of these herbal remedies, try to incorporate them into your daily or weekly routines. Drinking an infusion when you feel discomfort is helpful, but building a consistent habit can provide ongoing benefits:

• **Morning Ritual:** Start your day with a digestive support infusion to keep your stomach calm and balanced.
• **Evening Wind Down:** Make it a nightly ritual to enjoy a calming infusion before bed, helping you relax and improve your sleep quality.

Explanation of the categories

A. Digestive Health

Good digestion is essential for overall well-being, and these infusions are designed to help soothe common digestive issues such as bloating, indigestion, and IBS (Irritable Bowel Syndrome). Using a combination of carminative, anti-inflammatory, and soothing herbs, these blends can bring comfort to your digestive system, reduce discomfort, and support gut health.

B. Menstrual and Hormonal Balance

This section focuses on infusions that can support women during their menstrual cycle, alleviate PMS symptoms, and help balance hormones naturally. The herbs in these blends have been traditionally used to reduce cramps, calm mood swings, and promote overall hormonal balance, making them a natural choice for menstrual relief.

C. Calming and Stress Relief

In today's fast-paced world, managing stress is crucial. The infusions in this section are formulated to relax the body and mind, helping to reduce anxiety and promote better sleep. Whether you're unwinding after a long day or looking for a gentle way to calm your nerves, these blends will provide soothing relief.

Explanation of the categories

D. Immune Support and General Wellness

Boosting your immune system and maintaining general wellness is key to staying healthy year-round. These infusions contain herbs known for their immune-boosting, anti-inflammatory, and detoxifying properties. Whether you're looking to prevent illness or simply support your overall health, these blends will help you stay strong and balanced.

E. Energy and Focus

For those times when you need a natural energy boost without the jitters, the infusions in this section are formulated to enhance mental clarity and provide sustainable energy. These blends include herbs that support focus, memory, and alertness, making them perfect for your morning routine or whenever you need to power through the day.

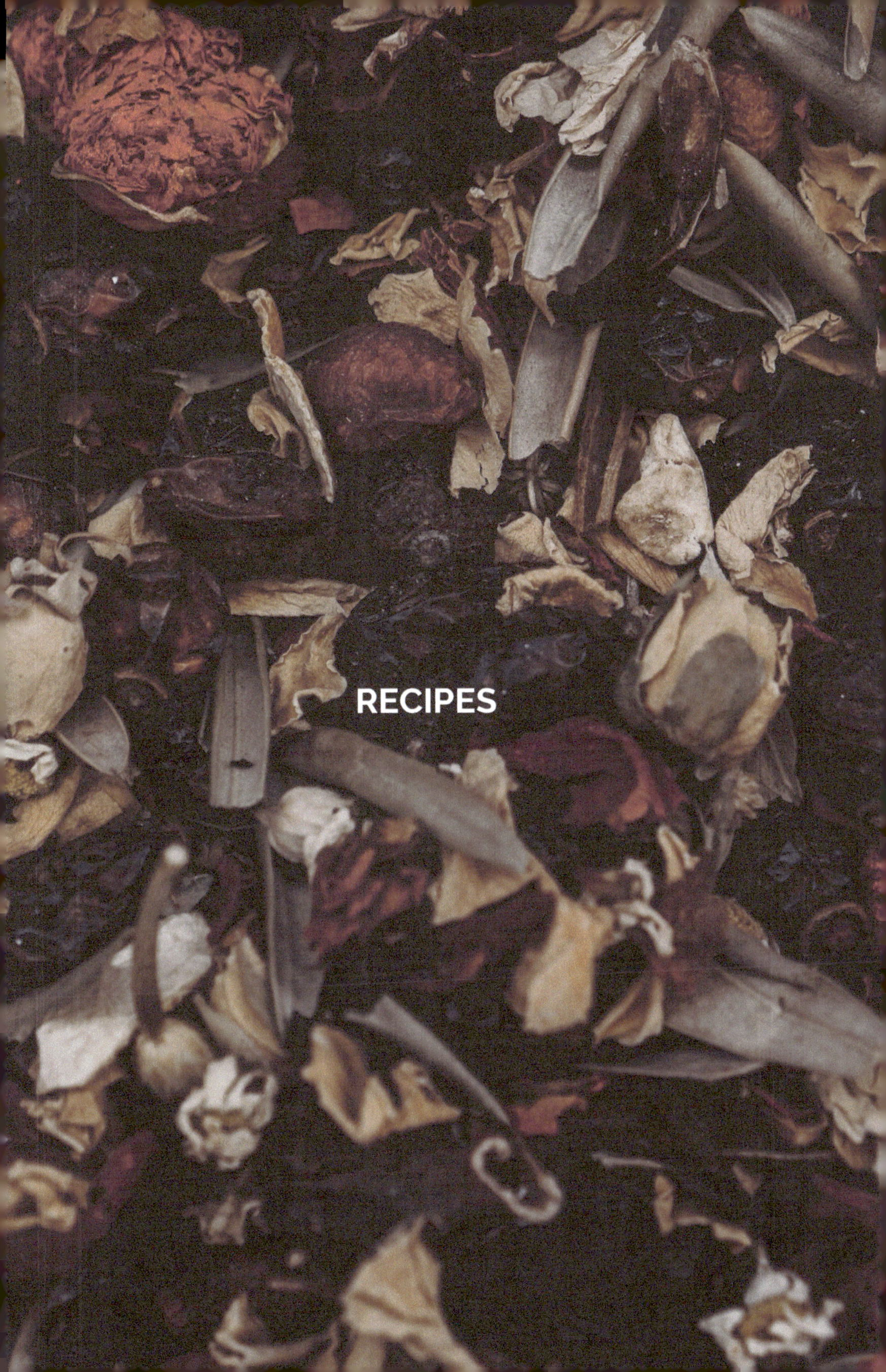
RECIPES

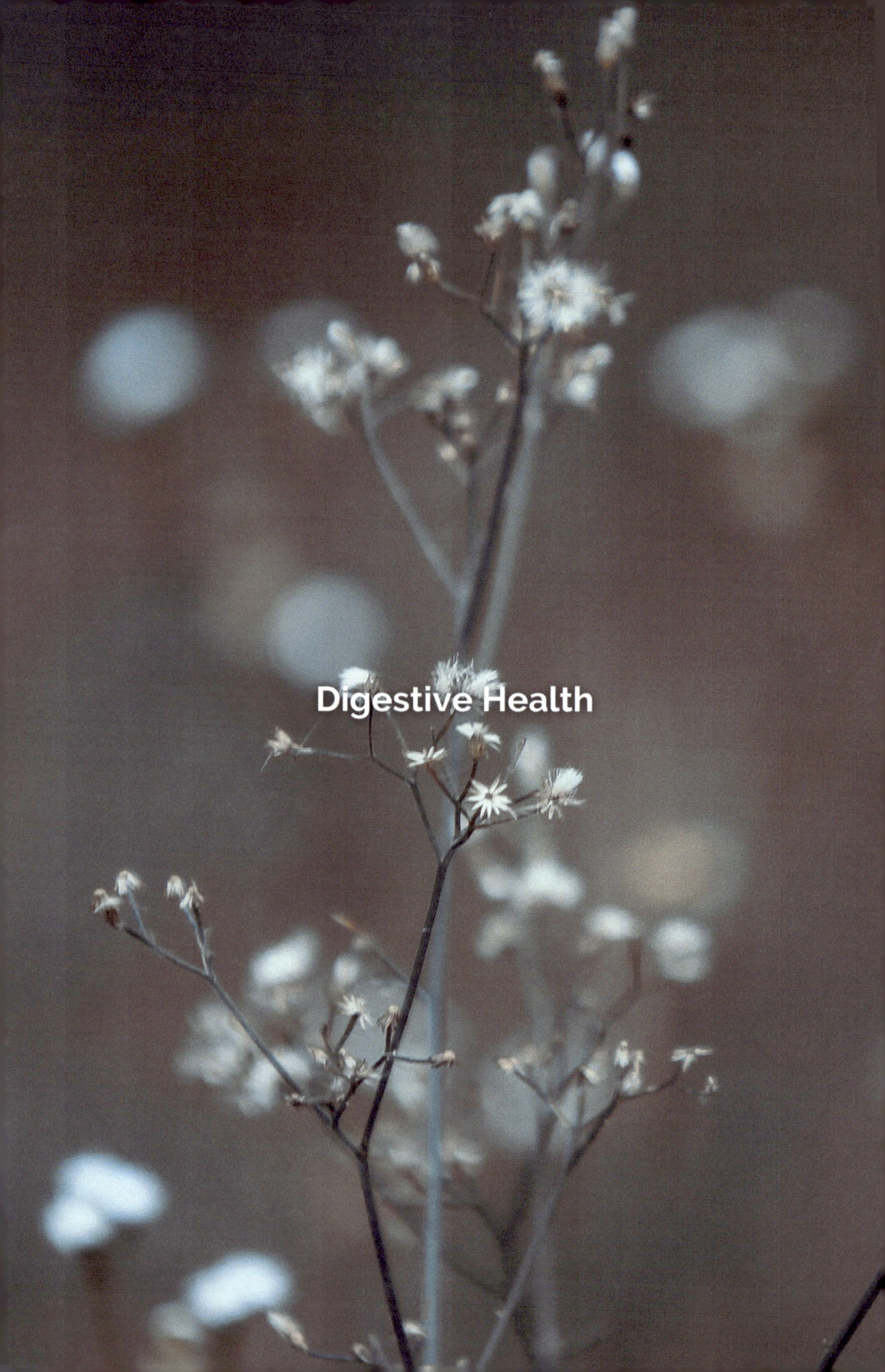

Digestive Health

Calming Stomach Tea

Category: Digestive Health
Servings: 1 cup

Ingredients:
 • 1 teaspoon Chamomile (Matricaria chamomilla)
 • 1 teaspoon Fennel (Foeniculum vulgare)
 • 1/2 teaspoon Linden (Tilia europaea)

Instructions:
 1. Bring 1 cup of water to a boil.
 2. Add chamomile, fennel, and linden to a teapot or cup.
 3. Pour the hot water over the herbs.
 4. Cover and let steep for 10-15 minutes.
 5. Strain and enjoy warm.

Additional Notes:
 • **Chamomile**: Calms the stomach and relieves digestive discomfort.
 • **Fennel**: Helps reduce gas and bloating.
 • **Linden**: Soothes the digestive tract.

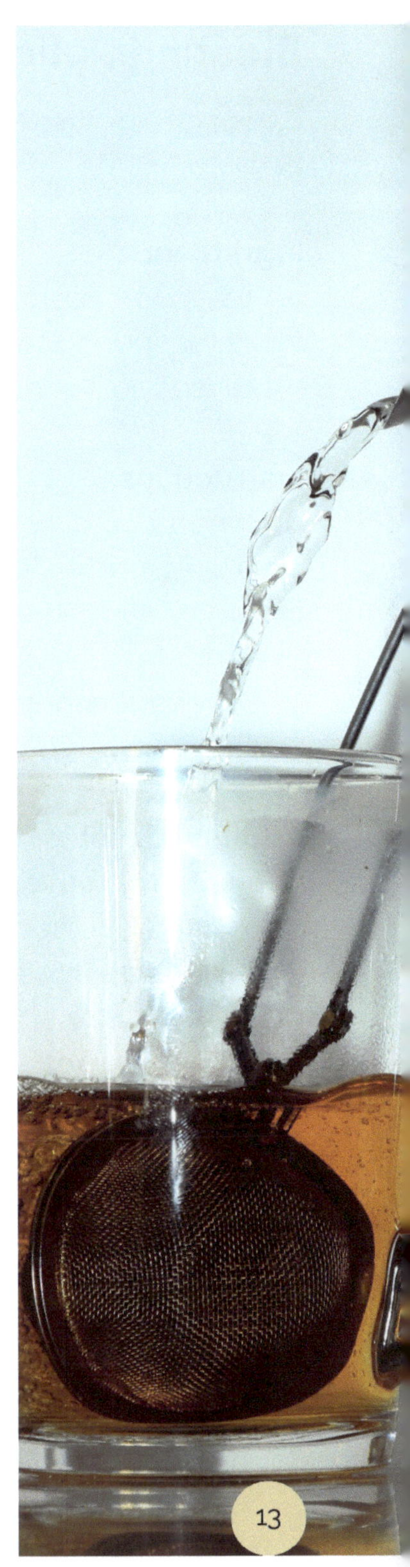

Bloating Relief Infusion

Category: Digestive Health
Servings: 1 cup

Ingredients:
- 1 teaspoon Raspberry leaves (Rubus idaeus)
- 1/2 teaspoon Star anise (Illicium verum)
- 1 teaspoon Dandelion root (Taraxacum officinale)

Instructions:
1. Bring 1 cup of water to a boil.
2. Add raspberry leaves, star anise, and dandelion root to a teapot or cup.
3. Pour the hot water over the herbs.
4. Cover and steep for 10-15 minutes.
5. Strain and enjoy after meals to relieve bloating.

Additional Notes:
- **Raspberry leaves**: Known for their ability to ease digestive discomfort and soothe the stomach.
- **Star anise**: Helps reduce bloating, aids digestion, and eases gas.
- **Dandelion root**: Promotes liver function and helps with water retention, easing bloating.

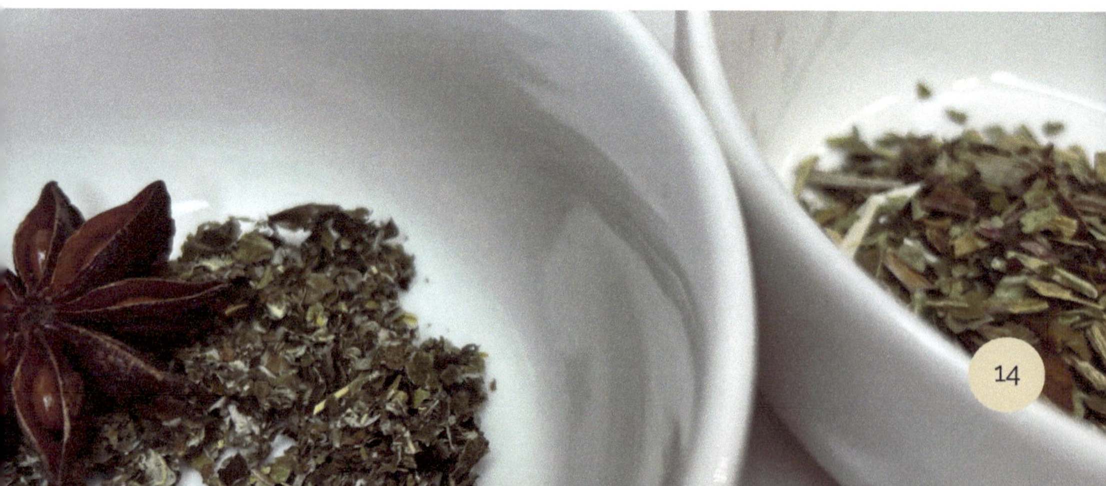

Gentle Gut Blend

Category: Digestive Health
Servings: 1 cup

Ingredients:
 • 1 teaspoon Sage (Salvia officinalis)
 • 1 teaspoon Calendula (Calendula officinalis)
 • 1/2 teaspoon Fennel seeds (Foeniculum vulgare)

Instructions:
 1. Boil 1 cup of water and pour it over the sage, calendula, and fennel seeds.
 2. Let the mixture steep for 10 minutes.
 3. Strain and enjoy this gentle blend to soothe and support digestion.

Additional Notes:
 • **Sage**: Balances and soothes the digestive system.
 • **Calendula**: Known for its anti-inflammatory properties, it helps with gut health and digestion.
 • **Fennel**: Reduces bloating and relieves digestive discomfort.

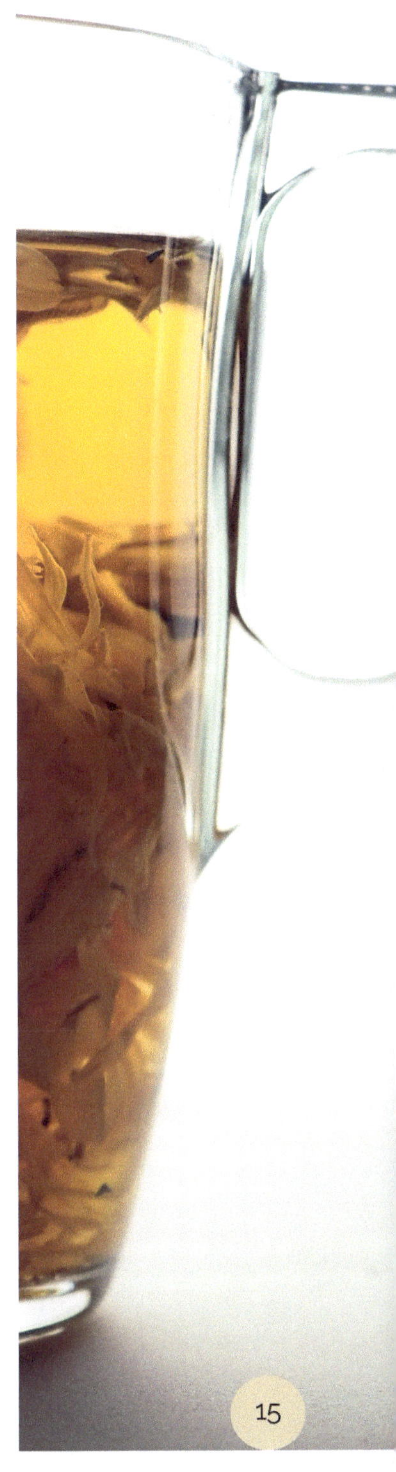

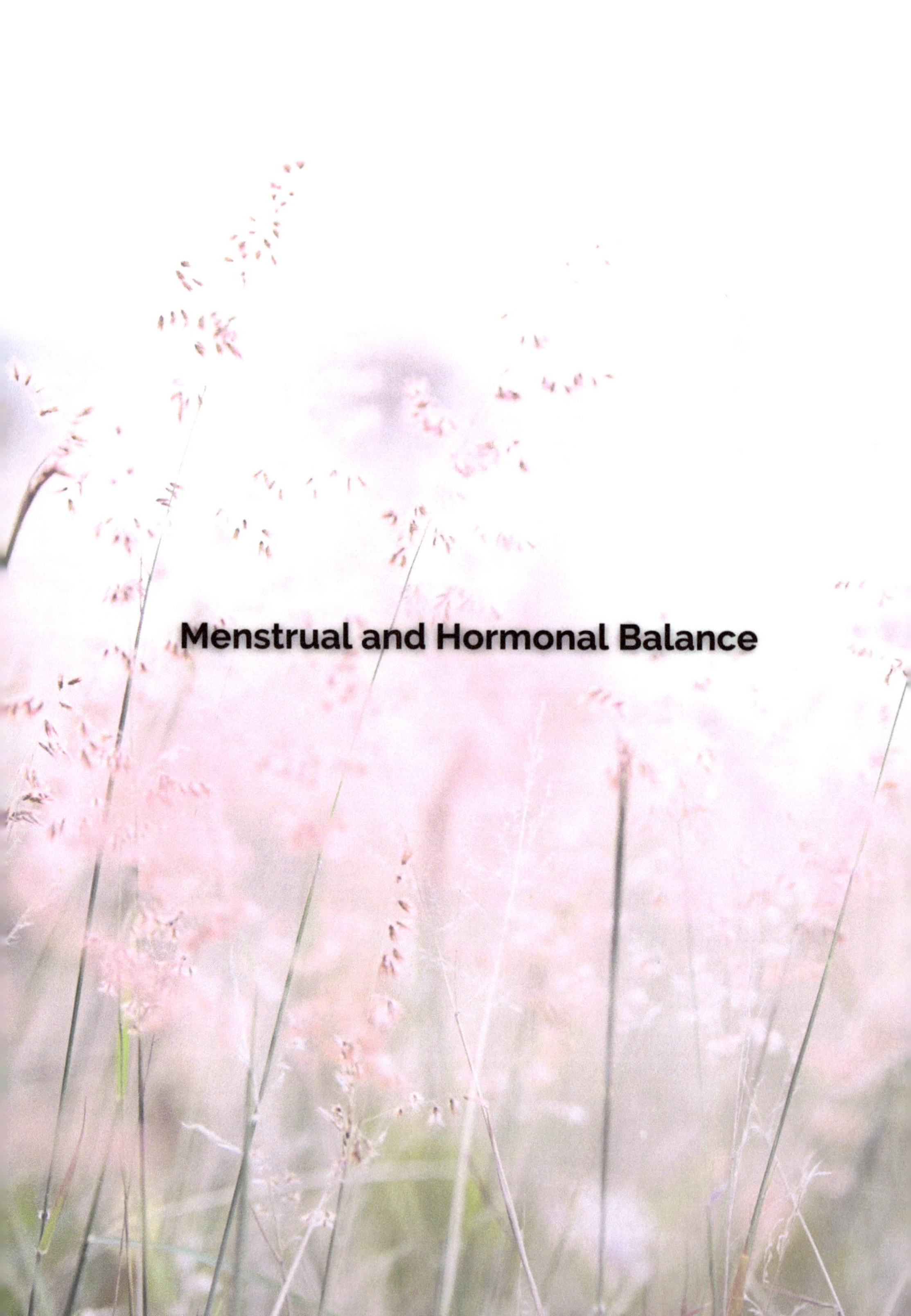
Menstrual and Hormonal Balance

Menstrual Relief Blend

Category: Menstrual and Hormonal Balance
Servings: 1 cup

Ingredients:
- 1 teaspoon Sage (Salvia officinalis)
- 1 teaspoon Chamomile (Matricaria chamomilla)
- 1/2 teaspoon Calendula (Calendula officinalis)

Instructions:
1. Boil 1 cup of water and pour over the sage, chamomile, and calendula.
2. Cover and let steep for 10-12 minutes.
3. Strain and drink warm to relieve menstrual discomfort.

Additional Notes:
- **Sage**: Helps balance hormones and reduces menstrual cramps.
- **Chamomile**: Soothes inflammation and helps relax the body.
- **Calendula**: Eases cramps and promotes healing.

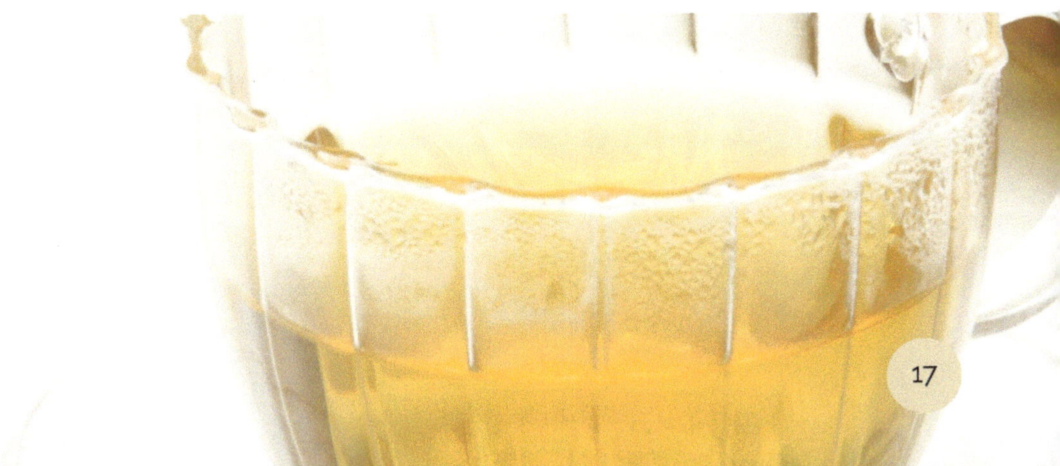

PMS Soothing Infusion

Category: Menstrual and Hormonal Balance
Servings: 1 cup

Ingredients:
- 1 teaspoon Raspberry leaves (Rubus idaeus)
- 1/2 teaspoon Valerian root (Valeriana officinalis)
- 1 teaspoon Linden (Tilia europaea)

Instructions:
1. Bring 1 cup of water to a boil.
2. Pour the boiling water over raspberry leaves, valerian root, and linden.
3. Steep for 10 minutes, covered.
4. Strain and enjoy warm for PMS relief.

Additional Notes:
- **Raspberry leaves**: Alleviates cramps and supports reproductive health.
- **Valerian root**: Calms anxiety and stress, promoting relaxation.
- **Linden**: Reduces mood swings and encourages restful sleep.

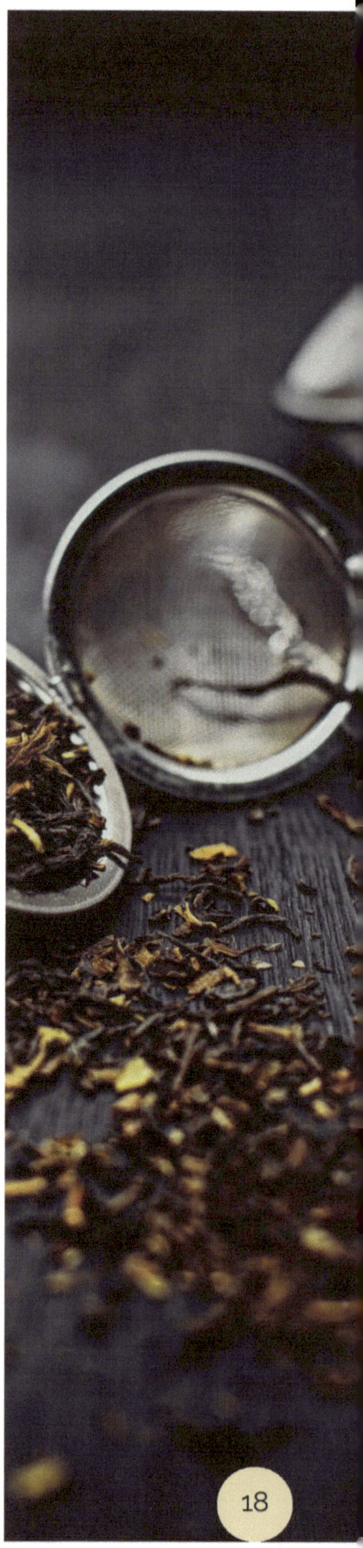

Hormone Harmony Tea

Category: Menstrual and Hormonal Balance
Servings: 1 cup

Ingredients:
- 1 teaspoon Ashwagandha (Withania somnifera)
- 1/2 teaspoon Sage (Salvia officinalis)
- 1 teaspoon Fennel seeds (Foeniculum vulgare)

Instructions:
1. Boil 1 cup of water and pour over ashwagandha, sage, and fennel seeds.
2. Let steep for 10-15 minutes, covered.
3. Strain and drink to help balance hormones and reduce stress.

Additional Notes:
- **Ashwagandha**: Known for its adaptogenic properties, helps balance hormones and reduce stress.
- **Sage**: Supports hormonal balance and soothes menstrual discomfort.
- **Fennel seeds**: Aids digestion and helps with hormonal-related bloating.

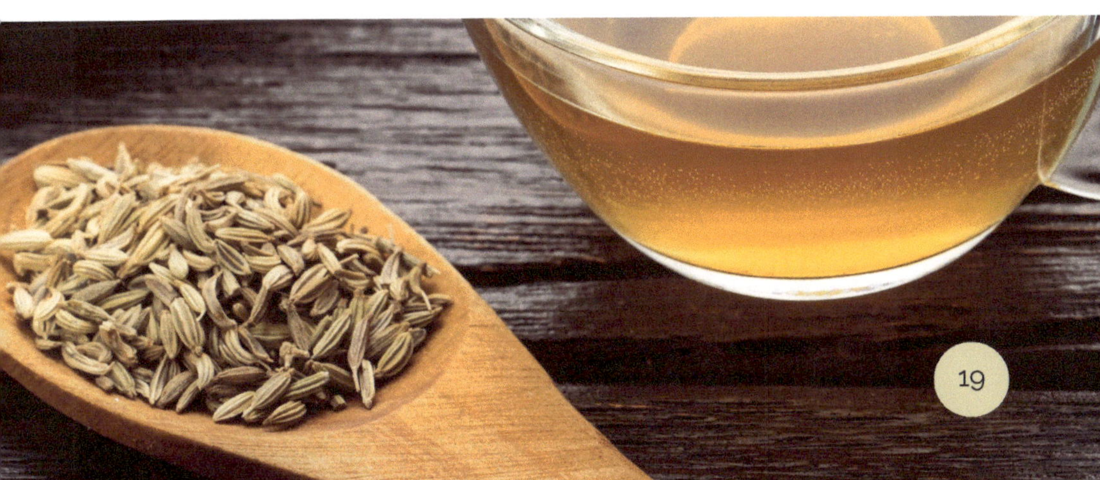

Calming and Stress Relief

Relaxing Evening Tea

Category: Calming and Stress Relief
Servings: 1 cup

Ingredients:
 • 1 teaspoon Valerian root (Valeriana officinalis)
 • 1 teaspoon Chamomile (Matricaria chamomilla)
 • 1 teaspoon Linden (Tilia europaea)

Instructions:
1. Bring 1 cup of water to a boil.
 2. Pour the boiling water over the valerian root, chamomile, and linden.
 3. Cover and let steep for 10-15 minutes.
 4. Strain and enjoy this calming tea before bed.

Additional Notes:
 • **Valerian root**: Helps relax the body and promote deep sleep.
 • **Chamomile**: Calms the mind and reduces anxiety.
 • **Linden**: Soothes and supports relaxation, perfect for winding down.

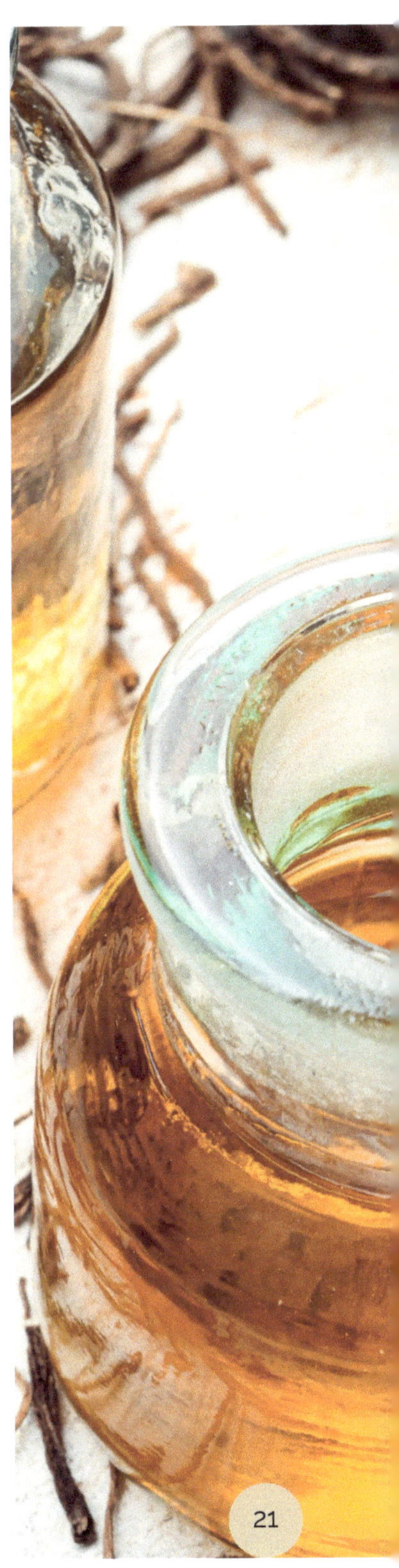

Stress Relief Blend

Category: Calming and Stress Relief
Servings: 1 cup

Ingredients:
- 1 teaspoon Ashwagandha (Withania somnifera)
- 1 teaspoon Lemon balm (Melissa officinalis)
- 1/2 teaspoon Chamomile (Matricaria chamomilla)

Instructions:
1. Boil 1 cup of water and pour it over the ashwagandha, lemon balm, and chamomile.
2. Cover and let steep for 10-12 minutes.
3. Strain and drink warm to help reduce stress and promote calm.

Additional Notes:
- **Ashwagandha**: A powerful adaptogen that helps reduce stress and balance cortisol levels.
- **Lemon balm**: Known for its calming effects on the nervous system.
- **Chamomile**: Gently relaxes both the body and mind.

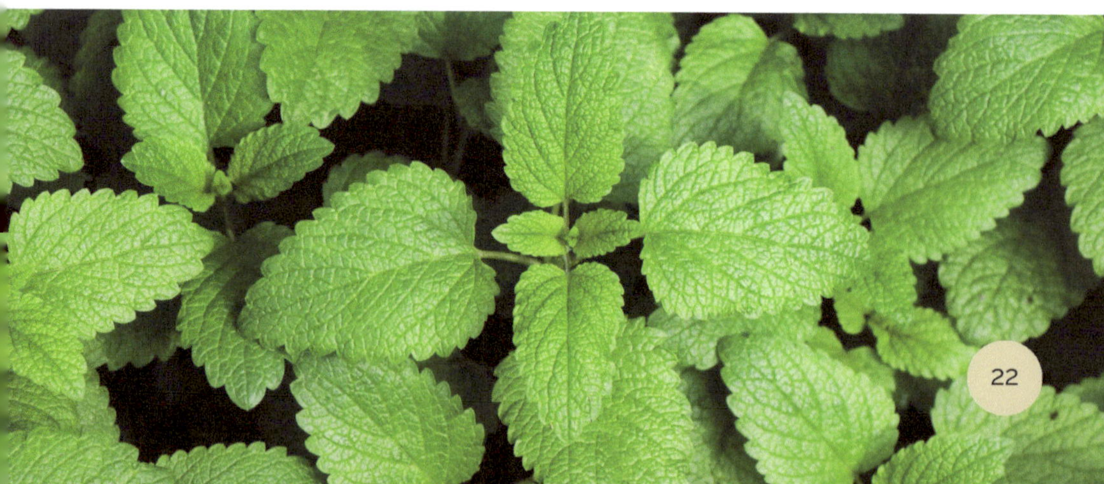

Calm Mind Tea

Category: Calming and Stress Relief
Servings: 1 cup

Ingredients:
 • 1 teaspoon Tila (Linden, Tilia europaea)
 • 1 teaspoon Rose petals (Rosa spp.)
 • 1/2 teaspoon Fennel seeds (Foeniculum vulgare)

Instructions:
 1. Bring 1 cup of water to a boil.
 2. Add the linden, rose petals, and fennel seeds to a teapot or cup.
 3. Pour the hot water over the herbs.
 4. Cover and let steep for 10-15 minutes.
 5. Strain and enjoy this soothing tea to calm the mind and reduce stress.

Additional Notes:
 • **Linden**: Soothes the nervous system and reduces tension.
 • **Rose petals**: Uplifts the mood and brings emotional balance.
 • **Fennel seeds**: Gently aids digestion and provides a calming effect.

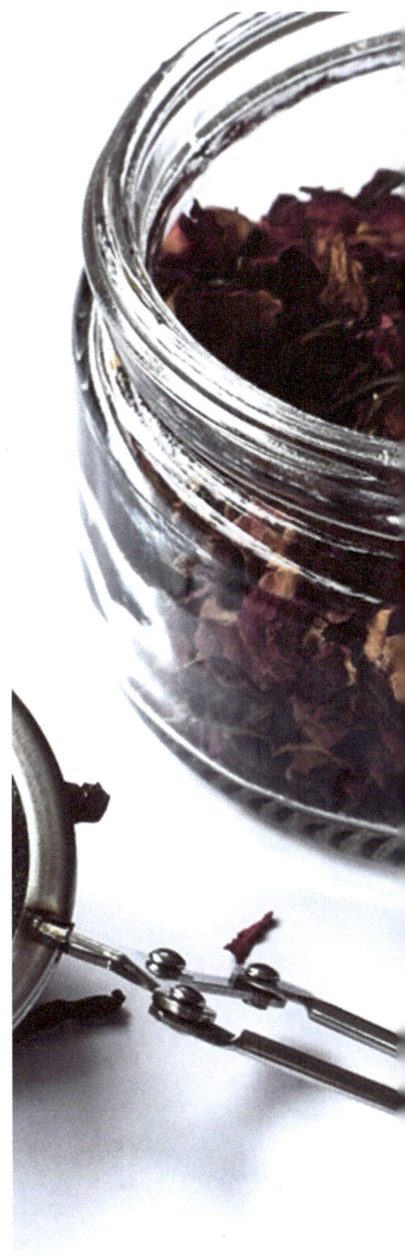

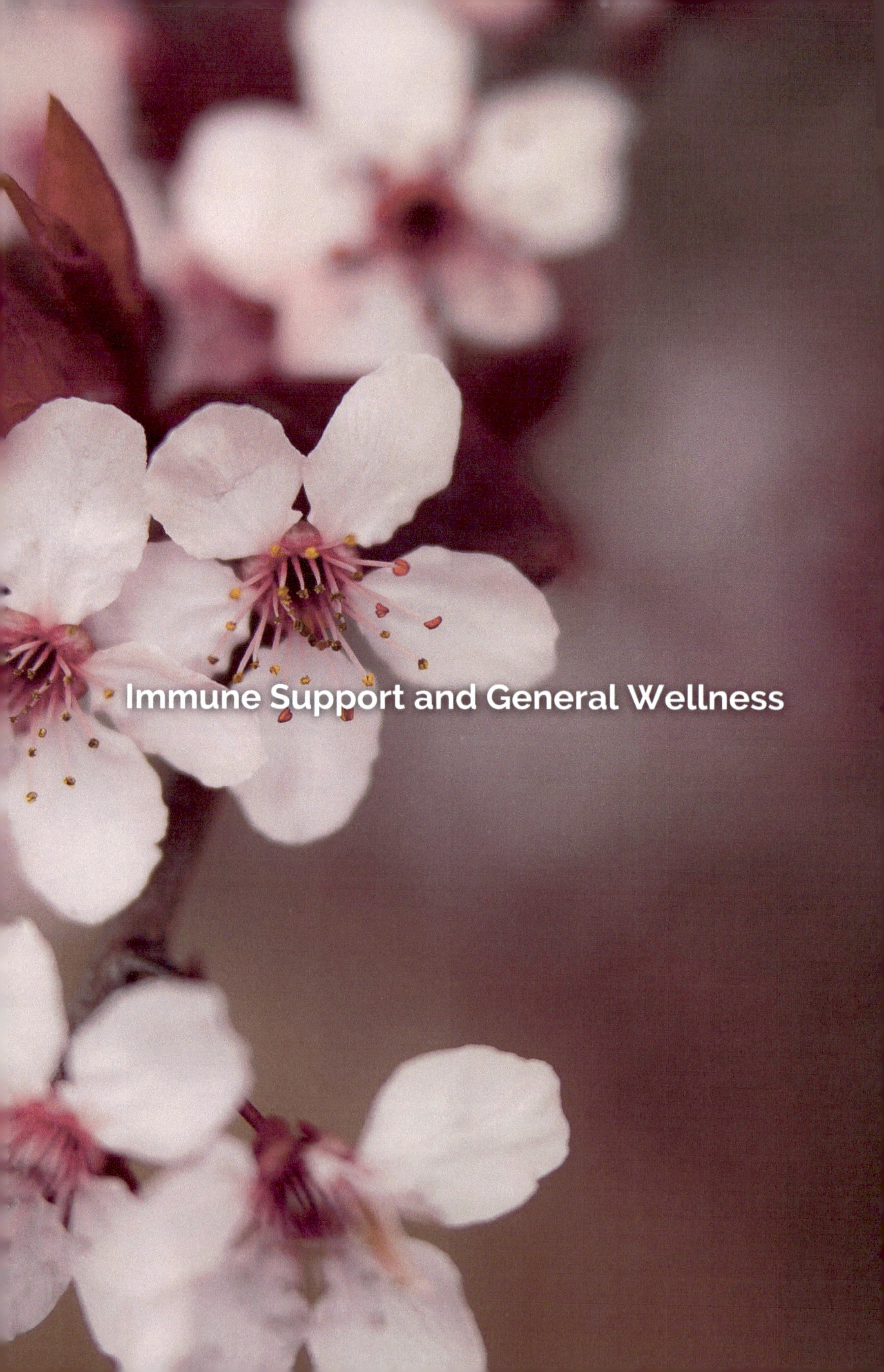
Immune Support and General Wellness

Immune Boosting Tea

Category: Immune Support and General Wellness
Servings: 1 cup

Ingredients:
• 1 teaspoon Sage (Salvia officinalis)
• 1 teaspoon Calendula (Calendula officinalis)
• 1/2 teaspoon Fennel seeds (Foeniculum vulgare)

Instructions:
1. Bring 1 cup of water to a boil.
2. Pour the hot water over the sage, calendula, and fennel seeds.
3. Cover and steep for 10-12 minutes.
4. Strain and drink to support your immune system and overall health.

Additional Notes:
• **Sage**: A potent herb for boosting immunity and fighting infections.
• **Calendula**: Known for its anti-inflammatory and healing properties.
• **Fennel seeds**: Helps support digestion and the immune system.

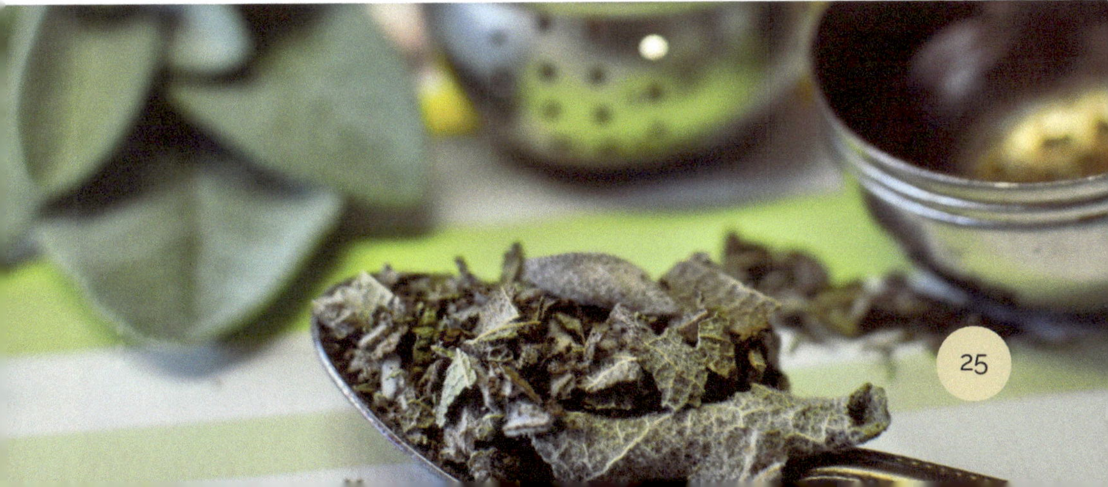

Cold and Flu Relief Infusion

Category: Immune Support and General Wellness
Servings: 1 cup

Ingredients:
 • 1 teaspoon Chamomile (Matricaria chamomilla)
 • 1/2 teaspoon Dandelion root (Taraxacum officinale)
 • 1 teaspoon Linden (Tilia europaea)

Instructions:
 1. Boil 1 cup of water and pour over the chamomile, dandelion root, and linden.
 2. Cover and let steep for 10-15 minutes.
 3. Strain and enjoy this soothing tea to ease cold and flu symptoms.

Additional Notes:
 • **Chamomile**: Reduces inflammation and supports restful sleep.
 • **Dandelion root**: Acts as a gentle detoxifier and supports liver function.
 • **Linden**: Soothes the throat and helps ease congestion.

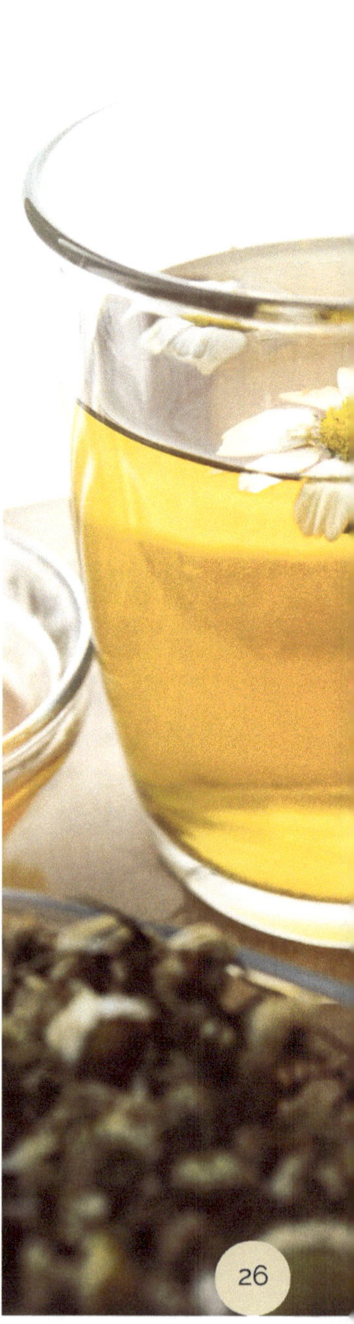

Wellness Support Blend

Category: Immune Support and General Wellness
Servings: 1 cup

Ingredients:
 • 1 teaspoon Rose petals (Rosa spp.)
 • 1 teaspoon Chamomile (Matricaria chamomilla)
 • 1/2 teaspoon Star anise (Illicium verum)

Instructions:
 1. Bring 1 cup of water to a boil.
 2. Add rose petals, chamomile, and star anise to a teapot or cup.
 3. Pour the hot water over the herbs.
 4. Cover and let steep for 10-12 minutes.
 5. Strain and enjoy this blend to promote overall wellness and vitality.

Additional Notes:
 • **Rose petals**: Provides antioxidants and uplifts mood.
 • **Chamomile**: Supports relaxation and boosts the immune system.
 • **Star anise**: Known for its antiviral and antimicrobial properties.

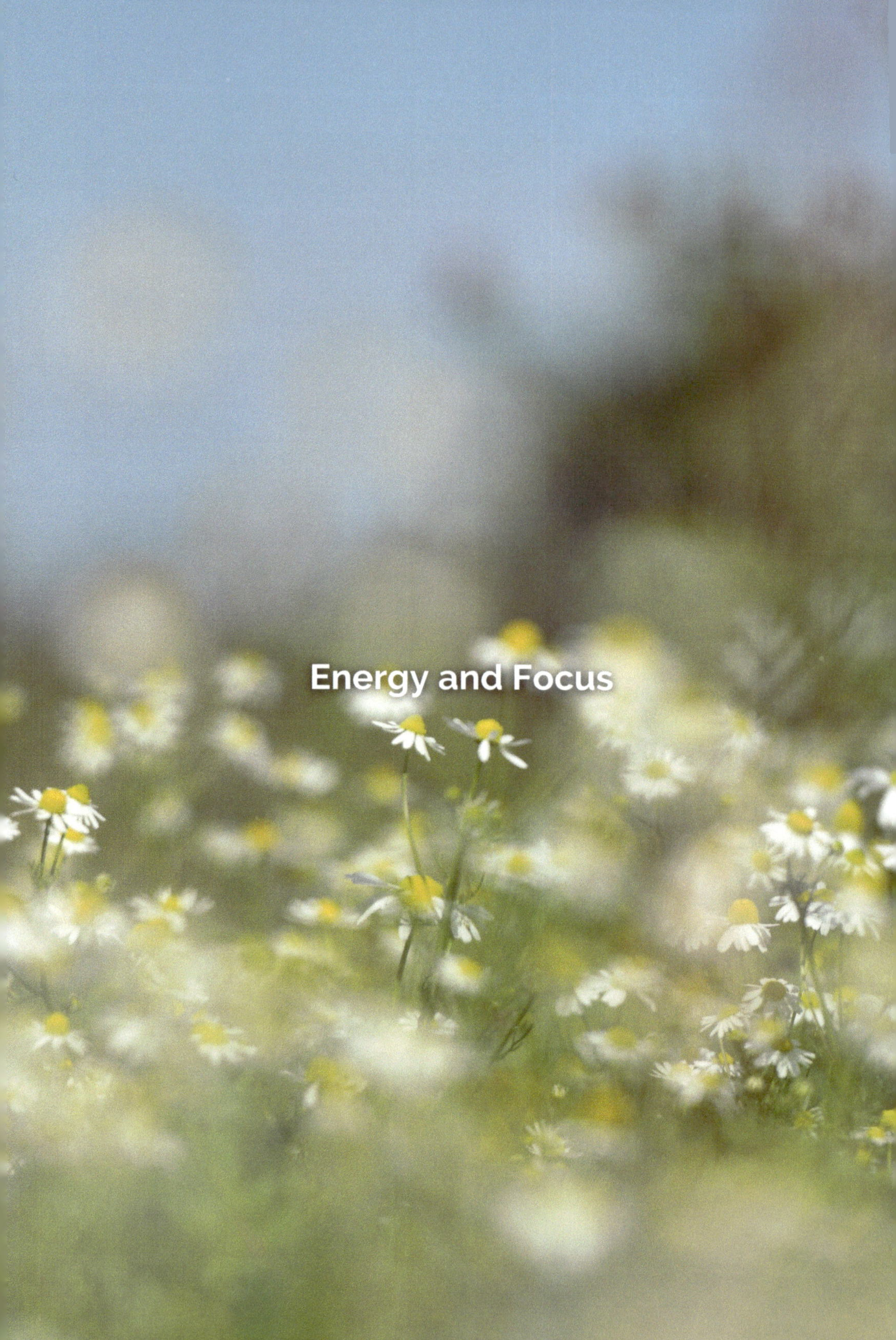
Energy and Focus

Morning Energy Boost Tea

Category: Energy and Focus
Servings: 1 cup

Ingredients:
 • 1 teaspoon Ashwagandha (Withania somnifera)
 • 1 teaspoon Sage (Salvia officinalis)
 • 1/2 teaspoon Fennel seeds (Foeniculum vulgare)

Instructions:
 1. Bring 1 cup of water to a boil.
 2. Pour the boiling water over the ashwagandha, sage, and fennel seeds.
 3. Cover and steep for 10-12 minutes.
 4. Strain and enjoy this tea in the morning to energize and support mental clarity.

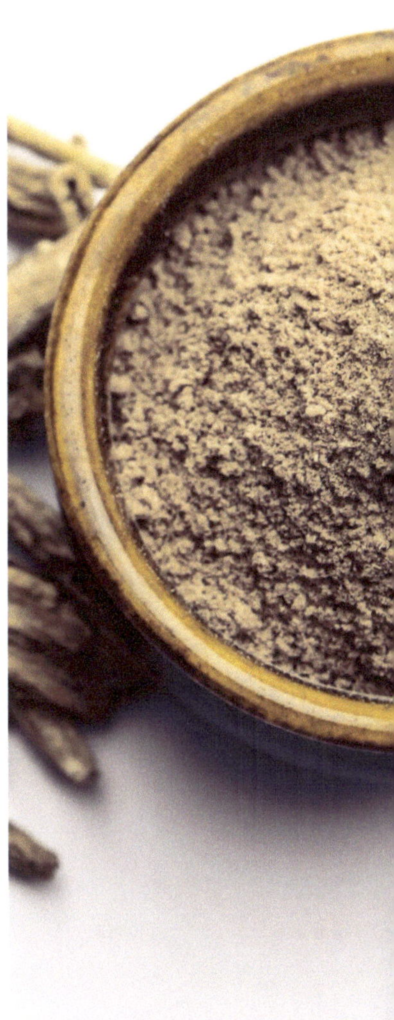

Additional Notes:
 • **Ashwagandha**: A powerful adaptogen that supports sustained energy and reduces stress.
 • **Sage**: Enhances mental focus and cognitive function.
 • **Fennel seeds**: Provides a gentle digestive boost and aids concentration.

Focus and Clarity Tea

Category: Energy and Focus
Servings: 1 cup

Ingredients:
- 1 teaspoon Lemon balm (Melissa officinalis)
- 1/2 teaspoon Dandelion root (Taraxacum officinale)
- 1 teaspoon Chamomile (Matricaria chamomilla)

Instructions:
1. Boil 1 cup of water and pour it over the lemon balm, dandelion root, and chamomile.
2. Cover and let steep for 10-15 minutes.
3. Strain and drink to improve mental clarity and support calm focus.

Additional Notes:
- **Lemon balm**: Calms the mind and enhances focus.
- **Dandelion root**: Boosts energy and supports liver function for mental clarity.
- **Chamomile**: Soothes the nerves, helping you stay focused.

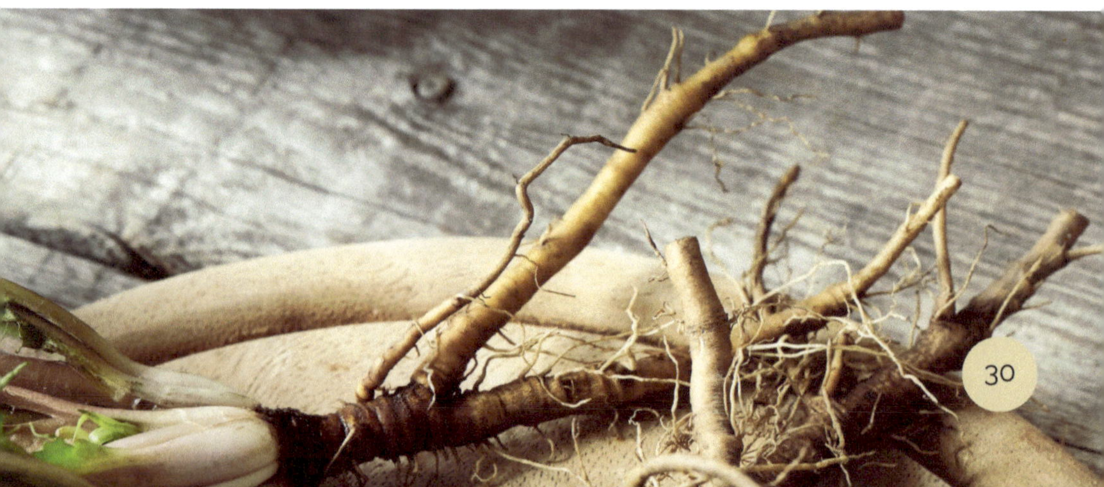

Revitalizing Tea

Category: Energy and Focus
Servings: 1 cup

Ingredients:
- 1 teaspoon Valerian root (Valeriana officinalis)
- 1 teaspoon Rose petals (Rosa spp.)
- 1/2 teaspoon Star anise (Illicium verum)

Instructions:
1. Bring 1 cup of water to a boil.
2. Add valerian root, rose petals, and star anise to a teapot or cup.
3. Pour the hot water over the herbs and cover.
4. Let steep for 10-12 minutes, strain, and enjoy for a refreshing energy boost.

Additional Notes:
- **Valerian root**: Helps reduce fatigue by supporting restful sleep.
- **Rose petals**: Provides antioxidants and enhances vitality.
- **Star anise**: Stimulates the mind and provides a natural energy boost.

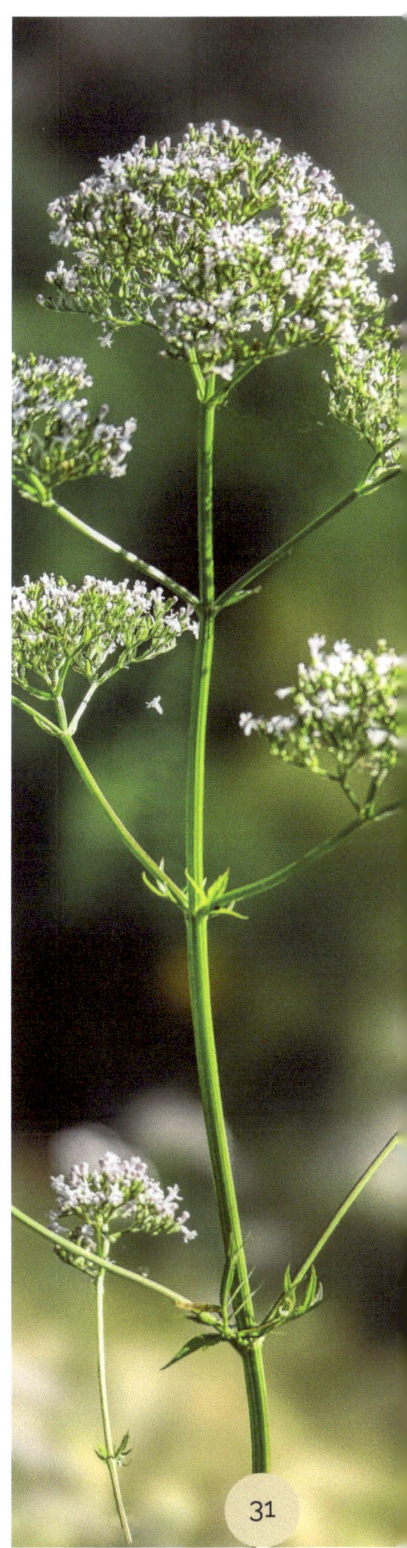

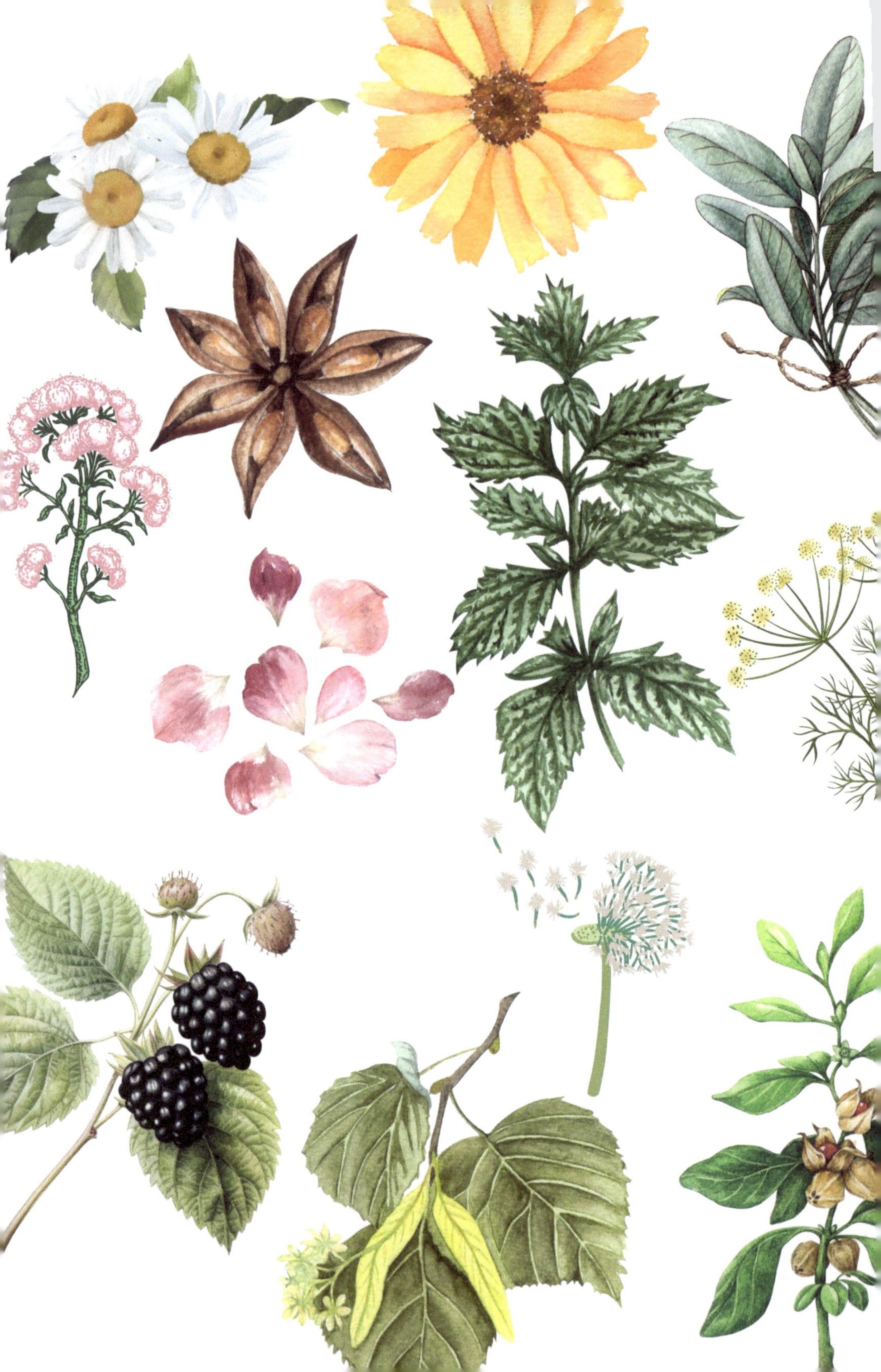

Herbs Section: Educational Information
Introduction to Medicinal Herbs

This section provides an overview of the most commonly used herbs in this book. You'll find their Latin names, primary benefits, and traditional uses. While these herbs are natural remedies, remember to consult a healthcare provider for specific conditions.

1. Sage (Salvia officinalis)

- **Benefits**: Hormonal balance, digestion support, and anti-inflammatory properties.
- **Traditional Uses**: Used for menstrual cramps, sore throats, and to enhance mental clarity.
- **Did you know?** Sage has been used for centuries in both culinary and medicinal practices for its antibacterial properties.

2. Chamomile (Matricaria chamomilla)

- **Benefits**: Calming, anti-inflammatory, and promotes relaxation.
- **Traditional Uses**: Widely known as a sleep aid and for easing digestive issues, especially bloating and cramps.
- **Did you know?** Chamomile is often called "the mother of the gut" because of its soothing effects on the digestive system.

3. Raspberry Leaves (Rubus idaeus)

- **Benefits**: Menstrual support, uterine health, and rich in vitamins and minerals.
- **Traditional Uses**: Often used by women to tone the uterus and ease menstrual discomfort.
- **Did you know?** Raspberry leaves are a common ingredient in pregnancy teas due to their ability to strengthen uterine muscles.

4. Ashwagandha (Withania somnifera)

- **Benefits**: Adaptogen, stress relief, and hormonal balance.
- **Traditional Uses**: Promotes energy, reduces stress, and supports overall hormonal balance.
- **Did you know?** Ashwagandha is one of the most important herbs in Ayurvedic medicine, revered for its ability to adapt to your body's needs.

5. Dandelion Root (Taraxacum officinale)

- **Benefits**: Detoxification, liver support, and digestive aid.
- **Traditional Uses**: Commonly used to promote healthy liver function and as a mild diuretic.
- **Did you know?** Dandelion is often considered a weed, but its roots and leaves are packed with vitamins and minerals.

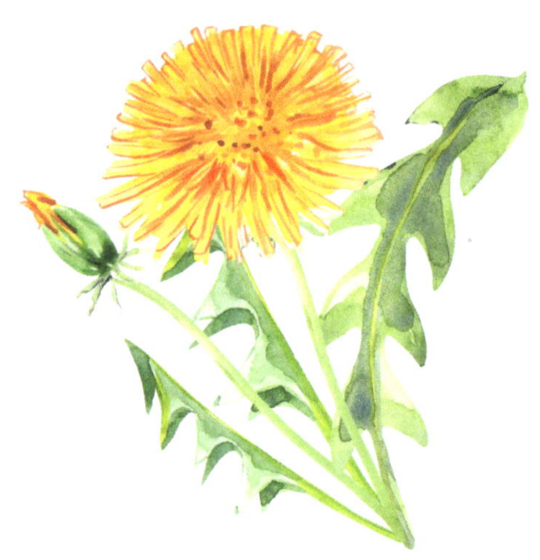

6. Valerian Root (Valeriana officinalis)

· **Benefits**: Sleep aid, anxiety relief, and muscle relaxation.
· **Traditional Uses**: Often used to treat insomnia and nervous tension.
· **Did you know?** Valerian root has been used since ancient Greece and Rome to treat insomnia and calm the nervous system.

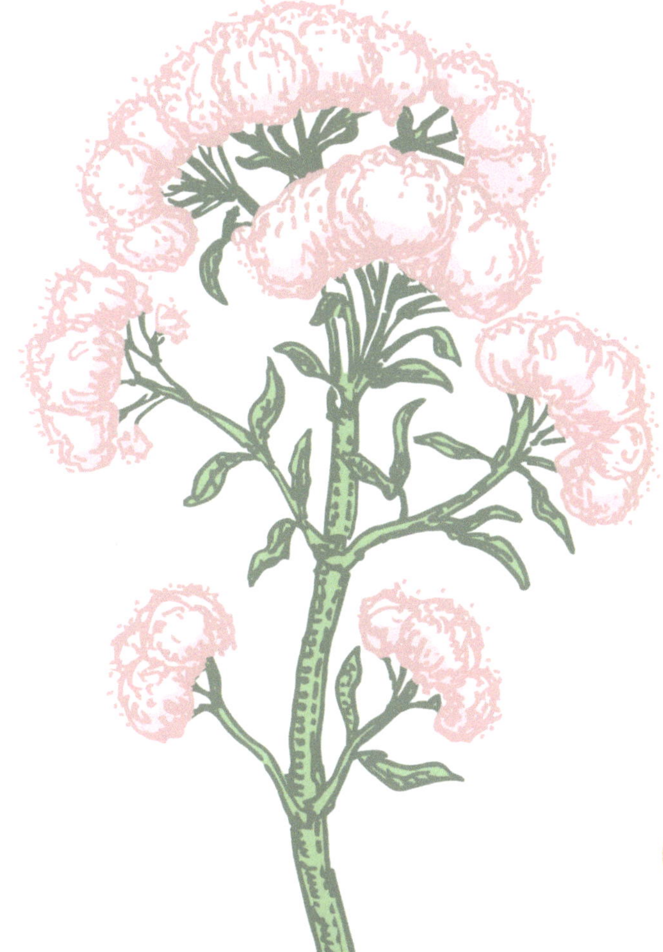

8. Linden (Tilia europaea)

- **Benefits**: Calming, sleep support, and stress relief.
- **Traditional Uses**: Used to calm anxiety, treat headaches, and promote relaxation.
- **Did you know?** Linden tea is often used as a natural remedy to help induce sleep in children.

9. Calendula (Calendula officinalis)

- **Benefits**: Skin health, anti-inflammatory, and wound healing.
- **Traditional Uses**: Often used topically to treat skin conditions, and internally for inflammation and menstrual cramps.
- **Did you know?** Calendula is sometimes referred to as "marigold" and is prized for its ability to soothe irritated skin.

10. Star Anise (Illicium verum)

- **Benefits**: Digestive aid, antimicrobial, and immune support.
- **Traditional Uses**: Often used to ease digestion, bloating, and as an antiviral remedy.
- **Did you know?** The shikimic acid found in star anise is a key ingredient in the production of some flu medications.

11. Rose Petals (Rosa spp.)

- **Benefits**: Mood enhancement, relaxation, and antioxidant-rich.
- **Traditional Uses**: Commonly used to uplift mood, reduce anxiety, and as a gentle digestive tonic.
- **Did you know?** Rose petals contain high levels of vitamin C and are often used to boost immune function.

12. Lemon Balm (Melissa officinalis)

- **Benefits**: Stress relief, cognitive support, and digestive aid.
- **Traditional Uses**: Known for its ability to reduce stress, enhance focus, and soothe the digestive system.
- **Did you know?** Lemon balm was called the "elixir of life" in the Middle Ages for its rejuvenating properties.

Daily Wellness Routines

Incorporating herbal infusions into your daily routine can be an easy and enjoyable way to support your overall well-being. Below, you'll find examples of how you can use the recipes from this book throughout the day to enhance energy, calm the mind, support digestion, and promote restful sleep.

Example Routine:

• **Morning**:
Start your day with an energizing blend like Morning Energy Boost Tea. The combination of ashwagandha and sage helps awaken your mind and body without the jitters of caffeine.
Recipe: Morning Energy Boost Tea (page 29)
• **Afternoon**:
For lunch, try a digestive infusion such as the Bloating Relief Infusion. It helps ease any bloating or discomfort, allowing you to stay light and energized through the day.
Recipe: Bloating Relief Infusion (page 14)
• **Evening**:
Wind down after a long day with a calming infusion like PMS Soothing Infusion or Calming Stomach Tea. These blends promote relaxation and help calm any premenstrual or daily stress.
Recipe: Calming Stomach Tea (page 13)
• **Before Bed**:
Enjoy a cup of Gentle Gut Blend before bed to promote digestion while you sleep and prevent discomfort overnight.
Recipe: Gentle Gut Blend (page 15)

Daily Wellness Routines

Routine 1: Calm and Balance (for Stressful Days)

A routine designed to keep you calm and grounded on days filled with stress and tension.

• **Morning**:
Start your day with Hormone Harmony Tea. This blend of sage and raspberry leaf helps balance hormones and promote a calm start to your day.
Recipe: Hormone Harmony Tea (page 19)

• **Mid-Morning:**
Sip on PMS Soothing Infusion to reduce any stress or anxiety that builds up as the day progresses. This infusion helps balance mood and calms your nerves.
Recipe: PMS Soothing Infusion (page 18)

• **Afternoon:**
As stress levels may peak in the afternoon, take a break with Calming Mind Tea. This tea contains valerian and chamomile to help ease mental tension and promote relaxation.
Recipe: Calming Mind Tea (page 23)

• **Evening:**
Before bed, have a cup of Relaxing Evening Tea to help transition into a peaceful night's sleep. This tea blend soothes your mind and body after a long day.
Recipe: Relaxing Evening Tea (page 21)

Daily Wellness Routines

Routine 2: Digestive Comfort (for Sensitive Stomachs)

Perfect for those who experience bloating, indigestion, or discomfort throughout the day.

• **Morning:**
Start your day with Gentle Gut Blend. This soothing combination of fennel, calendula, and chamomile gently supports digestion after breakfast.
Recipe: Gentle Gut Blend (page 15)

• **Late Morning:**
Mid-morning, enjoy Bloating Relief Infusion to ease any discomfort caused by meals or stress. The infusion is designed to reduce bloating and calm the digestive system.
Recipe: Bloating Relief Infusion (page 14)

• **Afternoon:**
After lunch, sip on Calming Stomach Tea to help promote digestion and prevent any heaviness or discomfort from meals.
Recipe: Calming Stomach Tea (page 14)

• **Evening:**
Wind down with a cup of Relaxing Evening Tea, perfect for calming the stomach and reducing any indigestion before bedtime.
Recipe: Relaxing Evening Tea (page 21)

Daily Wellness Routines

Routine 3: Energy Boost and Mental Clarity (for Busy or Long Days)

Ideal for days when you need to stay focused, energized, and alert throughout the day.

 • **Morning:**
Kickstart your day with Morning Energy Boost Tea, a blend of ashwagandha, sage, and dandelion to awaken your senses and enhance mental clarity.
Recipe: Morning Energy Boost Tea (page 29)
 • **Mid-Morning:**
For an extra boost of focus, sip on Focus and Clarity Tea, which combines valerian and rosemary for mental alertness and sustained concentration.
Recipe: Focus and Clarity Tea (page 30)
 • **Afternoon:**
In the mid-afternoon slump, have a cup of Revitalizing Tea to recharge your energy and prevent burnout. This blend supports long-lasting energy without the crash of caffeine.
Recipe: Revitalizing Tea (page 31)
 • **Early Evening:**
After work, sip on Calming Mind Tea to gently reduce stress while maintaining focus for any evening tasks.
Recipe: Calming Mind Tea (page 23)

Herb Storage and Preparation Tips

To make the most of your herbal infusions, it's important to properly store and prepare the herbs. Here are some tips to help you preserve the quality of your herbs and brew the perfect infusion.

Storage Tips:

- **Airtight Containers**: Store your herbs in airtight glass jars to preserve their potency. Avoid plastic containers, as they can affect the taste and quality.
- **Keep Away from Light**: Store your herbs in a dark, cool place. Exposure to sunlight can degrade their medicinal properties.
- **Label and Date**: Always label your jars with the name of the herb and the date you purchased or harvested it. Most herbs will maintain their potency for up to 1 year.

Infusion Preparation:

- **Boiling Water**: Use fresh, filtered water and bring it to a boil. For delicate herbs like chamomile or rose petals, let the water cool slightly before pouring over the herbs.
- **Steeping Time**: The average steeping time is 10-15 minutes, but this can vary based on the herb. For roots and tougher herbs, allow more time (up to 20 minutes).
- **Use a Cover**: Always cover your tea while steeping to keep the beneficial oils and aromas from evaporating.

Frequently Asked Questions (FAQ)

Here are some common questions and concerns about using herbal infusions. Remember, herbal remedies are a complement to a healthy lifestyle, and it's always best to consult a healthcare professional if you have any medical concerns.

1. How long does it take for an infusion to work?
  • Infusions typically take effect within 20-30 minutes, depending on the herb and your body's response. Some herbs, like those for digestion, work quickly, while others, like adaptogens, may need to be consumed regularly for long-term benefits.

2. Can I combine different herbs in one infusion?
  • Yes! Many herbs work synergistically, enhancing each other's benefits. For example, you can combine chamomile with fennel for both calming and digestive support. However, start with small amounts to ensure the blend agrees with you.

3. Is it safe to drink infusions every day?
  • Most herbs used in this book are safe for daily use, but it's important to rotate your blends to prevent overexposure to certain compounds. Some herbs, like dandelion root, should be taken in moderation as they have diuretic effects.

Frequently Asked Questions (FAQ)

4. Can I drink infusions during pregnancy or breastfeeding?

• Some herbs are safe during pregnancy, like raspberry leaf, which supports uterine health. However, always consult your doctor before taking any herbs during pregnancy or while breastfeeding.

DIY Herbal Remedies

Herbs aren't just for drinking! Many of the herbs featured in this book can be used for topical remedies or even bath blends. Here are a few simple ways to use herbs outside of the teapot.

1. Calendula Skin Tonic:

 • **Ingredients**: 1 tablespoon calendula petals, 1 cup boiling water.
 • **Instructions**: Steep the calendula petals in boiling water for 15 minutes. Let it cool, strain, and use it as a gentle skin toner or for soothing minor skin irritations.

2. Chamomile and Rose Bath Soak:

 • **Ingredients**: 1/2 cup chamomile, 1/2 cup rose petals.
 • **Instructions**: Place the herbs in a muslin bag or cheesecloth. Add to your warm bathwater and let soak for 15-20 minutes to relax and soothe your skin.

3. Sage and Fennel Hair Rinse:

 • **Ingredients**: 2 teaspoons sage, 1 teaspoon fennel seeds, 2 cups boiling water.
 • **Instructions**: Steep the sage and fennel in boiling water for 20 minutes. After shampooing, use this infusion as a final rinse to add shine and stimulate scalp health.

Seasonal Tea Blends

Herbs are seasonal gifts from nature, and adjusting your infusions to the seasons can provide specific support for what your body needs throughout the year. Here are some suggestions for seasonal herbal blends.

Summer Refreshment

- **Ingredients**: 1 teaspoon fennel, 1 teaspoon lemon balm, 1/2 teaspoon rose petals.
- **Instructions**: Steep for 10-12 minutes and enjoy iced for a refreshing summer drink that cools the body and aids digestion.

Autumn Immunity Blend

- **Ingredients**: 1 teaspoon sage, 1/2 teaspoon calendula, 1/2 teaspoon star anise.
- **Instructions**: Steep for 10-15 minutes and drink warm to support the immune system as the weather cools down.

Winter Warming Infusion

- **Ingredients**: 1 teaspoon chamomile, 1/2 teaspoon dandelion root, 1 teaspoon fennel seeds.
- **Instructions**: Steep for 12-15 minutes and sip slowly to promote digestion and keep warm during colder months.

Glossary of Herbal Terms

Below are definitions of some common herbal terms used throughout this book, to help you better understand the language of natural remedies.

Adaptogen: A natural substance that helps the body adapt to stress and promotes balance.

Diuretic: An herb that promotes the production of urine, helping the body expel excess water and toxins.

Antioxidant: A compound that inhibits oxidation and combats free radicals, which can damage cells.

Tonic: An herb or remedy that strengthens and revitalizes the body, often focusing on a specific system like the digestive or immune system.

Table of Contents

Table of Contents